MAXINE ROSALER

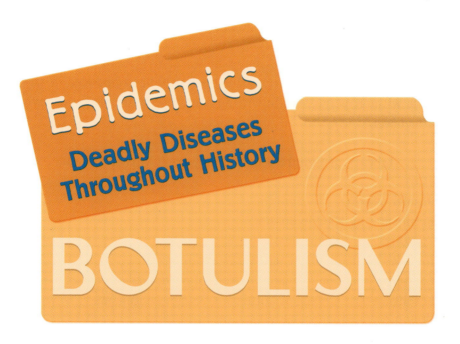

Epidemics
Deadly Diseases
Throughout History

BOTULISM

T 25382

The Rosen Publishing Group, Inc.
New York

Published in 2004 by The Rosen Publishing Group, Inc.
29 East 21st Street, New York, NY 10010

First Edition

Library of Congress Cataloging-in-Publication Data

Rosaler, Maxine.
Botulism / by Maxine Rosaler.
    v. cm. — (Epidemics)
Includes bibliographical references and index.
Contents: Botulism in history—Modern outbreaks—Types of botulism—The science of botulism—Battling botulism.
ISBN 0-8239-4197-3 (libr. bdg. : alk. paper)
1. Botulism—Juvenile literature. [1. Botulism. 2. Food poisoning. 3. Diseases.] I. Title. II. Series.
RC143 .R674 2003
614.5′125—dc21

                                                    2002152420

Manufactured in the United States of America

Cover image: A colorized magnification of *Clostridium botulinum*

CONTENTS

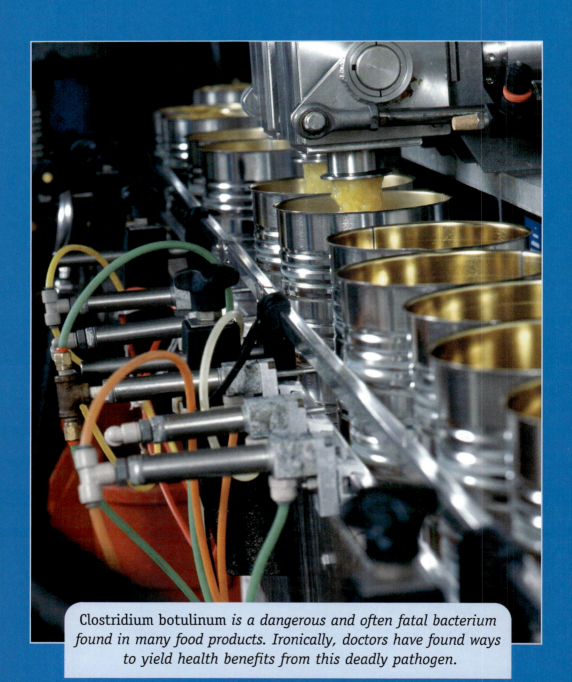

Clostridium botulinum *is a dangerous and often fatal bacterium found in many food products. Ironically, doctors have found ways to yield health benefits from this deadly pathogen.*

INTRODUCTION

Stay away from swollen cans of food! We are cautioned by everyone from our mothers to the Centers for Disease Control and Prevention (CDC). If we fail to heed that warning, the consequences can be dire: we might come down with botulism, a very rare and deadly disease.

Botulism is caused by a bacterium (plural: bacteria) called *Clostridium botulinum (C. botulinum* for short). *C. botulinum* can make people sick, often killing them, by producing a deadly toxin called botulinum toxin. Botulinum toxin is one of the most powerful poisons found in nature. It is colorless, odorless, and tasteless, and it works by paralyzing the nerves of its victim. Between twelve and thirty-six hours after swallowing the poison, the victim's mouth becomes dry and the person has trouble swallowing. The person's speech becomes unclear. He or she feels weak. As the poison continues to do its work, the victim experiences double vision, vomiting, severe diarrhea, and a muscle paralysis that gets worse over time. The paralysis usually starts with the eyes and face, and then moves downward to the throat, chest, arms, and legs. Finally, when the lungs become paralyzed, the victim can no longer breathe and ultimately dies.

The amount of botulinum toxin it takes to do this kind of damage is incredibly small. One gram of it is enough to kill a million people. The fact that so little of it can do so much harm makes this powerful toxin a popular weapon for bioterrorists. A Japanese religious cult planned to spray botulinum toxin in the Tokyo subways in the 1990s. The Iraqi dictator Saddam Hussein stockpiled 10,000 liters of it, planning to place it on missiles to be used in warfare.

Yet this same deadly poison is used by doctors to ease the symptoms of stroke and people suffering from muscular dystrophy. It is even used as a beauty treatment, helping to erase the signs of age. This is the dual nature of one of the deadliest bacteria known to humankind.

1

BOTULISM IN HISTORY

Botulism is older than recorded human history. When game was plentiful, our prehistoric ancestors saved up extra meat to help them through the lean times. Then, as now, food left to itself spoiled quickly, and anthropologists say our ancestors used some of the same preservation methods that are still used today by contemporary hunter-gatherer societies. They wrapped food in animal skins and animal organs, cured it with smoke, and then dried it. During the winter, they would bury the food in the ground, which served as a rudimentary refrigerator, allowing the food to freeze.

Most of the time these methods continue to work well, but they can lead to botulism if they are done improperly. The chances are that human beings have suffered from botulism for thousands of years.

Sausage Disease

The first botulism outbreak historians know of occurred in 1793 in the town of Wildbad, Germany. Thirteen people shared a meal of blood sausages, which was a favorite local dish. The sausages were prepared by washing out pig intestines and then stuffing them with blood and various spices. They were then tied at the ends, boiled briefly in water, smoked, and stored at room temperature for weeks at a time.

Most of the time, blood sausages could be eaten without any ill effects, but everyone who partook of this particular feast became very sick soon afterward. They vomited, their speech thickened, and some of them became partially paralyzed. The paralysis tended to become worse as time went on. In the end, six people died.

As a result, a local medical officer and physician named Justinus Kerner was sent to find out what had happened. Kerner was unable to conclude what had made the sausages so deadly, but he made some interesting observations that turned out to be useful to scientists who researched the causes of botulism

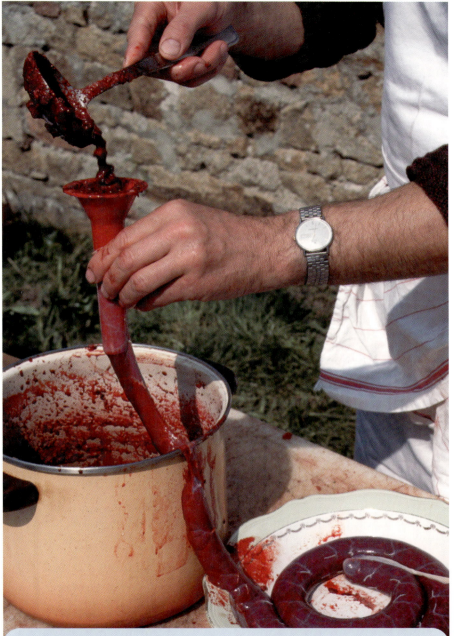

The first recorded case of botulism occurred in Germany during the eighteenth century and involved the consumption of blood sausage, the popular European dish pictured here.

many years later. For one thing, he noted that sausages didn't become poisonous if air pockets were present in their casings. He also noticed that the sausages that were housed in the larger casings were more apt to become poisonous. Finally, he noted that only the boiled sausages became poisonous.

To prove once and for all that it was the sausages that had caused the illness, Kerner went so far as to experiment on himself. He extracted a fluid from the sausages, which he called *wurstgift* (German for sausage poison), and injected it into his own body. He carried on with this dangerous experiment until he came down with enough of the symptoms to prove his point. Kerner went on to collect information about many other similar cases of food poisoning and published his findings in 1820. As a tribute to Kerner, for many years botulism was known as Kerner's disease.

The Rise of Bacteriology

Even for a researcher as determined as Kerner, there was a limit to what could be learned in his day about the poison. We know now that botulism is caused by bacteria, and no one knew about bacteria in the late eighteenth and early nineteenth centuries. In fact, at that time, no one understood that germs could cause infectious diseases. So little was known about germs in those days that surgeons did not even bother to wash their instruments between operations.

However, by the time the next major outbreak of botulism occurred, more than a hundred years later, many advances had been made in the science of medicine. The outbreak occurred in 1895 in Ellezelles, Belgium, among a group of amateur musicians. Thirty-four people became sick and three died as a result of this outbreak. As in the earlier outbreak, it was obvious that food—in this case, ham—was the culprit. Thanks to the discoveries made during the previous century, this time it was possible to learn a great deal more about what had caused the outbreak.

In the years since Kerner had published his findings, a revolution had occurred in medicine. In the 1860s and 1870s, Louis Pasteur and Robert Koch, working separately, had each developed the theory that diseases were caused by germs. This is what is commonly known as the germ theory of disease. This groundbreaking theory included the idea that infectious illnesses were spread by microscopic organisms that could multiply very quickly once they were inside the body.

In 1876, Koch proved that a bacterium called *Bacillus anthracis* caused the disease anthrax. In essence, Koch's work helped prove that the germ theory of disease was true. Three years later, in 1879, Pasteur developed a vaccine for a form of cholera that attacked chickens. Pasteur's chicken cholera vaccine showed that giving animals a weakened, harmless version of a microbe that causes a particular disease can help them to fight off infection from that same microbe should they ever become exposed to it. Pasteur later used this theory to develop a vaccine to protect people against rabies. Pasteur's work with the chicken cholera vaccine lent further support to the germ theory of disease.

At first the ideas of Pasteur and Koch were met with great skepticism. There were many other competing theories of disease, the most popular one being that disease was caused by "bad air." Some scientists simply would not believe the germ theory. In an attempt to disprove the theory, one prominent scientist asked Robert Koch for a sample of cholera bacteria and then swallowed it. The scientist didn't get sick, but this proved only that he had, as we would say now, a strong immune system. Eventually the medical community came around to accepting Koch's and Pasteur's theories.

By the end of the nineteenth century, the germ theory was generally accepted. Surgeons were washing their hands before operations and soaking their instruments in disinfectants to kill germs. Governments in Europe and the United States were working

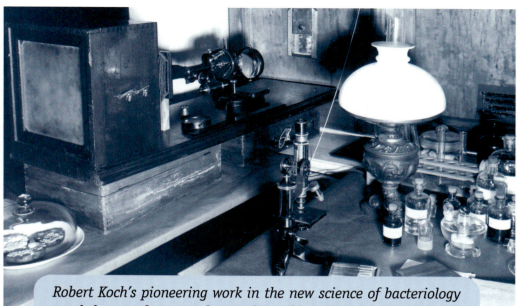

Robert Koch's pioneering work in the new science of bacteriology paved the way for an understanding of botulism. His laboratory in Wollstein, Germany, is pictured here.

to improve public sanitation, since germ-infested food and water were now recognized as major causes of illness. It was expected that each infectious disease would turn out to have its own microbe, and scientists were at work hunting for each of them, one by one.

Botulism Gets Its Name

By 1895, bacteriology (the study of bacteria) was a separate area of medical specialization. The incident of the poisoned ham was investigated by Emile Pierre Marie van Ermengem, professor of bacteriology at the Medical School of Ghent. Van Ermengem started his investigation using the new tools of bacteriology that had been developed by Robert Koch. These included methods of isolating and growing bacteria, the use of test animals, and various special dyes that made bacteria easier to see under a microscope. He gave bits of the ham to lab animals and watched as they came down with the deadly illness. From the ham and from the spleen of one of the people who had died from eating it, he discovered the bacteria that causes botulism and the poison that causes its symptoms. Van Ermengem's research established the basic facts of botulism as we know them today.

Van Ermengem gave the name "botulism" to the illness caused by the poisoned food, and he gave the name *Bacillus botulinus* to the bacterium that is the illness's root cause. "Bacillus" is the word that bacteriologists use to describe any bacterium that is shaped like a rod. *Botulinus* means "sausage" in Latin, and van Ermengem used the word because he was convinced that the disease Kerner described back in 1820 was caused by the same bacterium that had harmed the amateur musicians in Belgium.

Spores

Not only did van Ermengem give botulism its name, but he unlocked an important mystery concerning

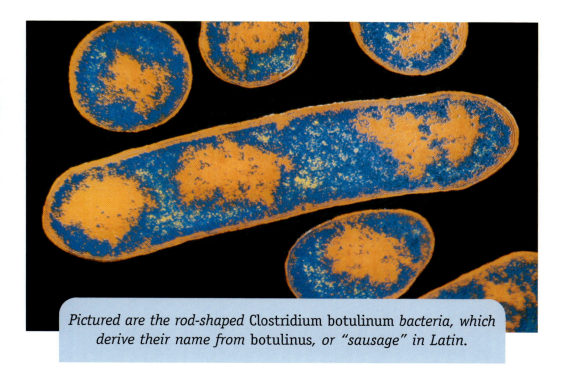

Pictured are the rod-shaped Clostridium botulinum *bacteria, which derive their name from* botulinus, *or "sausage" in Latin.*

the way it spreads. Earlier, Robert Koch had discovered that some bacteria can change their form. When they need to survive harsh living conditions, such as when there isn't enough food or moisture, they can dry out and produce thick, tough protective coats. In this form the bacteria are called spores, and their tough outer coatings are called spore coats. Van Ermengem found that *C. botulinum* was one of these spore-forming bacteria.

As spores, the bacteria are inactive. They can't do anything except lie in wait for living conditions to improve. The spores, though, can wait around for amazingly long periods of time. Spores have been

The state of Alaska has had one of the highest rates of food-borne botulism poisoning in the world. Most of the outbreaks occur among Native Americans who live in coastal villages in the western and southeastern parts of the state. This is because they follow a tradition of preserving food in a way that can sometimes lead to botulism, a method that in fact may have been causing botulism for thousands of years.

Early Arctic explorers reported that natives sometimes died from food poisoning. From descriptions that have been found about how the natives preserved food in those days, modern physicians suspect that these deaths were caused by botulism.

For example, Edward William Nelson, an American ethnographer, described the preparation of specially fermented foods that were called "stink foods," which he saw during a visit to the coastal villages of northwest Alaska from 1878 to 1881. "In the district between the Yukon and Kuskokwim," he wrote, "the heads of king salmon, taken in the summer, are placed in small pits in the ground surrounded by straw and covered with turf. They are kept there during the summer and in the autumn have decayed until even the bones have become the same consistency as the general mass. They are taken out and kneaded in a wooden tray until they form a pasty compound and are eaten as a favorite dish."

With these preservation methods, the Alaskans were, without knowing it, using harmless microbes to ferment the salmon heads. (Europeans have been making cheese and wine for thousands of years using essentially the

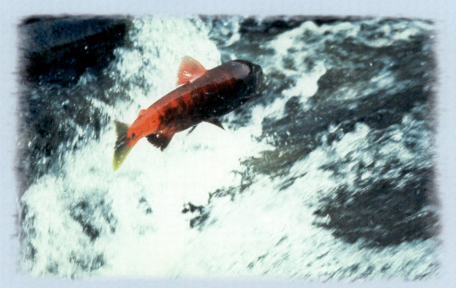

Pictured is a salmon as it travels upstream to spawn. When these fish are caught and stored for food, the potential exists for botulism contamination.

same methods.) Since the Alaskans didn't know that microbes were fermenting their food, they also didn't know that dangerous bacterial spores could infect the salmon heads, and that the result could be deadly.

Salmon heads treated this way are still a traditional delicacy in many coastal Alaskan villages. The problem is even worse today than it used to be because now Alaskan villagers often use glass and plastic jars, buckets, and plastic bags to store the salmon heads. These containers are airtight. Since oxygen kills the bacteria that cause botulism, using airtight containers can increase the risk of botulism.

known to stick around for thousands of years. When they finally find themselves again in a place that provides warmth, moisture, and the food they need, they absorb water, shed their protective coats, grow new cell walls, and become active, and deadly, again.

The ability of *C. botulinum* to form spores is an important factor in why it is able to spread. While the bacterium in its active form can be easily killed by regular cooking temperatures (five minutes at 212°F, or 100°C, thirty minutes at 176°F, or 80°C), the bacteria in spore form are able to resist these temperatures. Today we know that a temperature of at least 248°F (120°C), sustained for thirty minutes, is required to be sure of killing the bacteria that cause botulism.

Van Ermengem also proved that *C. botulinum* is anaerobic, which means that it cannot grow in the presence of oxygen. The fact that the bacterium that causes botulism is anaerobic is the reason why its original name, *Bacillus botulinus*, was later changed to *Clostridium botulinum*. *Clostridium* refers to the anaerobic group of bacteria.

Although oxygen kills *C. botulinum*, it does not kill *C. botulinum* spores. This was an important fact to know when van Ermengem set out to figure out why only the sausages that had been boiled developed botulism. Van Ermengem discovered that not only had the boiling not been hot enough to kill the spores, but it indirectly helped them turn back into active bacteria. Instead of killing the spores, the boiling drove the oxygen out of the sausages, creating the oxygen-free environment in which these anaerobic bacteria thrive.

2

THE SCIENCE OF BOTULISM

The oldest form of life on Earth, bacteria have been in existence for more than 3.5 billion years, and for the first billion years they had the planet all to themselves.

Bacteria, including the microbe that causes botulism, are neither plant nor animal, although they do have some of the features of both. They reproduce by a process known as binary fission. The word "fission" means "split," and the word "binary" means "two." In other words, bacteria reproduce by splitting in two.

Bacteria tend to reproduce very quickly, as often as once every twenty minutes. Using the method of binary fission, one bacterium becomes two, two become four, four become eight, until what was just one bacterium a few days before is now billions.

As a group, bacteria are essential to life on Earth. They perform the function of decomposing organic matter such as leaves and other living remains and turning it into soil that is usable by plants. Without bacteria, we would have no plants, and without plants, we would have no animals.

However, while most bacteria are beneficial or harmless, a few, such as the bacteria that cause botulism, are among humanity's deadliest enemies. Despite their small numbers, the bad bacteria are responsible for some of the most devastating diseases known.

A Deadly Strategy

Like all living things, bacteria need to find food and reproduce. Over the course of billions of years, each different kind of bacteria has developed its own strategy for survival. The diseases that some bacteria cause are part of their survival strategy.

Take the bacterium *Vibrio cholerae*, which causes cholera, a disease that has killed many millions of people in Europe and Asia over the course of history. One of the major symptoms of cholera is diarrhea. This diarrhea is *Vibrio cholerae*'s way of spreading itself, since *Vibrio cholerae* lives not only in people who have the disease, but also in their feces. In the days before good public sanitation, drinking water would often get contaminated with waste products. By drinking the contaminated water, healthy people would unknowingly take the bacteria into their bodies and become sick. Thus, the disease would continue to spread in a vicious cycle.

C. botulinum has developed a different but equally effective way to move about and find food. The method is a poison that works in a way that allows the bacteria to get around a serious weakness it has. Unlike some other bacteria, *C. botulinum* isn't very good at infecting live animals and human beings. As long as we're alive, our immune systems—the body system that fights off infections—are quite effective at killing *C. botulinum* bacteria. In fact, most of us eat and breathe *C. botulinum* spores all the time without any ill effects.

To get around this problem, over time *C. botulinum* has developed a powerful weapon, the nerve poison known as botulinum toxin. This poison spreads in dead plants or animal matter. It kills many of those who make the mistake of eating it. When an animal is dead, its immune system no longer functions. Having no immune system to fight them, the bacteria are free to multiply inside the dead body.

From here, the bacteria can spread by one of two ways. When an animal dies, there is always the possibility that its body will be eaten by scavengers. If the body that the scavenger eats is infected with the *C. botulinum* bacteria, the scavenger will contract botulism. Eventually the scavenger dies, thereby becoming the next breeding ground for the bacteria. If no scavenger finds the corpse and it continues to decay in the soil, *C. botulinum* bacteria will then turn into spores and wait for wind or water to spread them to a moist, low-acid, oxygen-free environment where they can shed their spore coats and multiply.

How Botulinum Toxin Works

The botulinum toxin is a colorless, odorless, and tasteless protein that our digestive enzymes can't break down. It is small enough to pass through the lining of the digestive tract to be absorbed into the bloodstream, and from there it can travel throughout the body.

Botulinum starts to do its damage when its journey through the bloodstream carries it to the places where nerve endings meet muscle cells. Usually the nerve cells that tell muscles to work do so with the help of a chemical called acetylcholine. Botulinum keeps the nerve endings from releasing acetylcholine. As a result, the muscle doesn't move and the victim is paralyzed.

1793
Wildbad, Germany

A feast of home-made blood sausages leads to vomiting, paralysis, and death. Justinus Kerner investigates and develops the theory that the outbreak was caused by a naturally occurring poison.
13 sick, 6 dead.

1895
Ellezelles, Belgium

An improperly cured ham causes illness in a group of amateur musicians, leading Emile van Ermengem to discover the bacterium *C. botulinum*.
34 sick, 3 dead.

1904
Darmstadt, Germany

A batch of canned white beans leads to the discovery that *C. botulinum* can grow in vegetables and to the discovery of a new strain of the bacterium called type A.
21 sick, 11 dead.

1919
California
Outbreaks of botulism in several states are caused by commercially canned olives. 19 dead.

1920–1922
California
Outbreak in commercially canned spinach leads to a government investigation and the development of new procedures to prevent further outbreaks. 26 dead.

1971
New York and Israel
An incident involving a single batch of Bon Vivant brand vichyssoise leads to the destruction of millions of cans of soup. 3 sick, 1 dead.

1974
Pontiac, Michigan
Home-canned hot peppers served at a restaurant are contaminated. 59 sick.

2002
FDA approves use of Botox.

Once blocked by the toxin, the nerve endings are permanently unusable. The body can't repair them. However, the nerves themselves aren't dead and can still sprout new nerve endings, which is what they start to do if the victim survives the poisoning. As these new nerve endings begin to work, muscle movement starts to come back. Recovery from botulism poisoning can take months or years, depending on how bad the case was.

Most people stricken with botulism poisoning begin to show symptoms of it within eight to thirty-six hours. Their mouths become dry, they have trouble swallowing, their speech is slurred, and they feel weak. They begin to see double, to vomit, and to have severe diarrhea along with muscle paralysis, which gets worse over time. The paralysis usually starts with the eyes and face and continues down to the throat, chest, arms, and legs. Finally the lungs become paralyzed, which leads to death unless the victim is put on a mechanical ventilator, a breathing machine.

Where Botulism Occurs

Botulism spores are found in the soil and in plants and animals all over the world, so health experts believe that botulism poisoning occurs everywhere, at one time or another. Most of the cases that are reported, however, occur in modernized industrial countries that have excellent public health systems. This statistic is a little misleading, however. Industrialized societies probably do not suffer more botulism outbreaks than poor, underdeveloped countries. Rather, botulism outbreaks in underdeveloped countries go unreported.

In Europe, where reporting is generally good, Poland is known as the country with the highest levels of foodborne botulism. This was especially true during the 1970s and 1980s. In the worst year, 1982, there were 738 cases of botulism, 15 of which resulted in death. According to health experts, the reason that there have

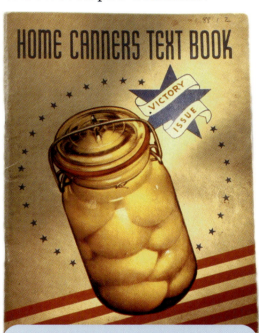

The Home Canners Text Book *offers advice on how to can food safely.*

been so many cases of botulism in Poland is that home canning is very popular there. While the majority of people who do home canning know how to do it safely, there are always a few people who

Botulinum toxin is one of the most poisonous substances known. One gram of botulinum toxin can kill more than one million people. Botulinum toxin is also very easy and cheap to obtain, which has made it attractive to terrorists or governments seeking a cheap weapon of mass destruction. It is so cheap and so destructive, like other biological weapons, it is sometimes called a "poor man's atomic bomb."

One terrorist group has already tried to use botulinum toxin in this way. On three separate occasions between 1990 and 1995, a Japanese cult named Aum Shinrikyo attempted to use botulinum toxin as a weapon of mass destruction. Cult members collected *C. botulinum* bacteria from soil in northern Japan and grew the toxin. They planned to release the poison into the air by spraying it in a crowded Tokyo subway, but after a change in plans they used sarin gas, a nerve poison, instead.

Unfortunately, larger and more sophisticated organizations have also investigated the possibility of using botulinum toxin as a weapon. One Japanese biological warfare group fed cultures of *C. botulinum* to prisoners in Manchuria in the 1930s. The United States biological weapons program produced botulinum toxin in World War II. Fearing that the Germans might be doing the same thing, the United States produced a million doses of botulinum vaccine for Allied troops preparing to invade Normandy on D-Day. In the end, however, botulinum toxin was not used during World War II. In the years that followed, many other countries conducted research into the possible use of botulinum toxin as a weapon.

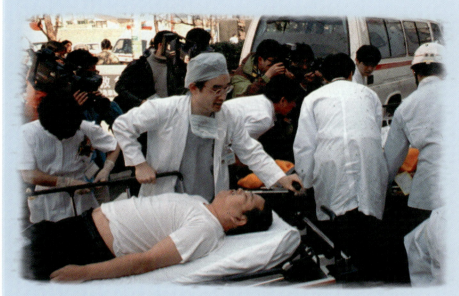

Some people fear that C. botulinum *might be used in biological attacks, such as the 1995 sarin gas attack in Tokyo, Japan, pictured here.*

The United States's research into the use of botulinum ultimately ended in 1970, and in 1972 the production of biological weapons was banned by the Biological and Toxin Weapons Convention (BWC). However, at least two of the signers of the pact, Iraq and the Soviet Union, continued to work on *C. botulinum* as a weapon. And with the breakup of the Soviet Union, many of the scientists who had worked on the Soviet biological weapons program went to work for other countries, including Iran, Iraq, North Korea, and Syria. Each of these countries has been listed by the U.S. government as "state sponsors of terrorism."

(Continued on page 30)

BOTULISM AND TERRORISM

(Continued from page 29)

Iraq is the country that has gone the furthest in trying to develop the botulinum toxin into a potential weapon. After the 1991 Persian Gulf War, a United Nations inspection team found that Iraq had produced 19,000 liters of botulinum toxin and had loaded 10,000 liters of it onto military weapons. This quantity of toxin is approximately three times the amount needed to kill every human being on Earth. It was loaded on specially designed missiles that had a range of 600 kilometers. Much of the toxin that Iraq produced is still unaccounted for.

don't, and so there will be more mistakes made in places where more canning is done.

After Poland, Italy is the European country that has had the most cases of botulism, followed by Germany, France, and Spain. Most of the cases are foodborne, as in Poland, and the culprit is usually something home-made, rather than a commercially processed food. The number of cases per year in these countries is far lower than in Poland, though. In Italy's worst year, 1990, there were fifty-four cases; in Germany's worst year, 1988, there were thirty-nine cases; in France's worst year, 1990, there were eleven cases; and in Spain's worst year, 1992, there were twelve cases.

Based on reports of occasional outbreaks, health experts believe that Asia is the continent in which

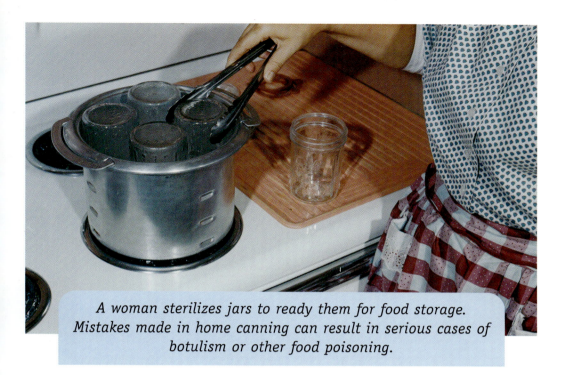

A woman sterilizes jars to ready them for food storage. Mistakes made in home canning can result in serious cases of botulism or other food poisoning.

botulism is most widespread and that the problem is the most serious in China. Botulism spores are often found in honey imported from China. This suggests that infant botulism—which is caused when babies consume food that contains botulism spores—may also be a problem in China, as it is in the United States. However, botulism in China is underreported, just as it is in poor, underdeveloped countries. So it is therefore difficult to confirm this assumption.

3

MODERN OUTBREAKS

For most of the twentieth century, botulism has been spread by a method of food preservation: canning.

When canning was first invented, the germ theory of disease had not yet been developed. It was believed that oxygen caused food to spoil and that canning worked by keeping oxygen out of the can. We now know that canning preserves food because the can's contents are sterilized when they are heated after the can has been sealed. Heating the can's contents kills the microbes that are already present in the food, and since the can is sealed, other microbes can't get at the food. When it's done correctly, canning is an excellent method of preventing food spoilage. It has also improved human nutrition by enabling people to preserve fruits, vegetables, and meats for long periods without drying, salting, or curing them.

Problems arise, however, when the can is not heated enough to kill the spores that cause botulism. As we now know, *C. botulinum* loves a moist, oxygen-free environment, especially, it has turned out, one that is low in acid, which is why low-acid foods like olives and spinach are especially prone to botulism. In the twentieth century, outbreaks of foodborne botulism caused by underheated cans led to a greater understanding of the risks associated with canning and botulism. Strict regulation of the canning process has made botulism in commercial canning rare. However, incidents involving home canning continue.

It is hard to prevent mistakes in home canning from occurring, since this is something that is done in so many different places by individuals and small groups. Government regulators don't have the means of imposing safety standards on individuals, as they do on businesses. They can't go into people's homes and inspect their kitchens, as they can go into the factories of commercial food producers to inspect them. Instead, regulators must content themselves with trying to educate people about safety standards and reminding home canners to make sure that their equipment is working properly. Despite

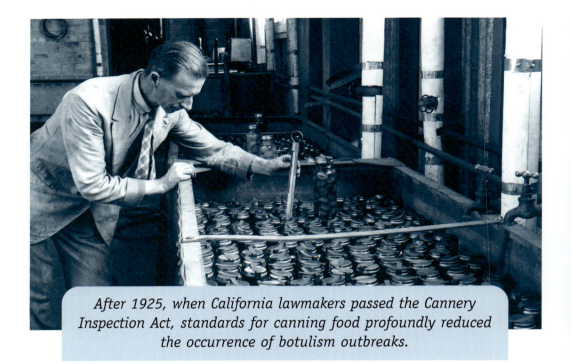

After 1925, when California lawmakers passed the Cannery Inspection Act, standards for canning food profoundly reduced the occurrence of botulism outbreaks.

regulators' efforts to educate people about the dangers, home canning is the most common cause of foodborne botulism.

The Great Can Scares

At first, scientists thought that only meat and fish could act as breeding grounds for botulism. But several years after Emile van Ermengem isolated the bacterium that causes botulism, it was found in other foods as well. In 1904, twenty-one people in Darmstadt, Germany, came down with cases of botulism that were caused by canned white beans. Eleven of the people who were sickened died. In this outbreak, a new strain of the bacterium was found—it was called type A botulism.

The problem of commercial canning causing botulism hit its worst point in the early 1920s in California. The state had by then become one of the world's largest producers of olives, which are the kind of low-acid foods that *C. botulinum* thrives in. In 1919, botulism that was caused by olives that had been commercially canned in California caused nineteen deaths across the nation. There were seven deaths in Ohio, five in Montana, and seven in Michigan. From 1920 to 1922, twenty-six deaths caused by botulism were linked to canned spinach produced in California, as well as four in Wyoming and four in California due to commercially produced canned olives.

Public health authorities were understandably alarmed by this, as were the canning companies, who feared they would soon be out of business if people started to become afraid of eating their products. In response to these outbreaks, canning associations in California directed a team of researchers to investigate the matter. Led by bacteriologist Karl F. Meyer, the team of researchers experimented with new canning methods that would prevent future outbreaks. Based on the recommendations of Meyer's team, state lawmakers formulated the California Cannery Act

What about the swollen and dented cans that mothers and many advice columns commonly remind families to throw away? Are these signs that the food contained in the damaged cans could cause botulism, and if so, why?

Swollen cans are certainly a bad sign. Many bacteria release gases when they grow and multiply, so a can swollen by the gases may indeed be a sign that the food inside has been contaminated, perhaps by *C. botulinum*. The CDC advises people to not even risk opening a can that appears swollen.

On the other hand, a dented can is not as likely to be as dangerous as a swollen can might be. Botulism by itself will not dent a can, but legend has it that at the turn of the century, unscrupulous merchants would bang on the swollen cans. Doing this redistributed the gas in the can, reducing the swelling and making them appear normal. Because of this, dented cans soon became as much a sign of contamination as the swollen ones. Today, however, merchants would not be likely to employ these kinds of tricky practices (for one thing, they'd be afraid of getting sued if they were ever found out), so a dent is most probably a sign that a can simply fell off the shelf. But dented cans should be avoided anyway, especially if there's a hole in them. These could be contaminated with all kinds of bacteria, *C. botulinum* included.

of 1925. The act required that products that could easily be contaminated with the *C. botulinum* bacteria be inspected at every step of the canning process. The act was so effective that it became a model for canning regulations worldwide. Since the act was put into place, contaminations at U.S. canneries have been extremely rare.

Bon Vivant Vichyssoise

Another outbreak occurred in 1971 in New York and Israel. The *C. botulinum* bacteria were found in a batch of the Bon Vivant brand of vichyssoise (vee-she-SWAZ), which is a French soup. The soup is traditionally served cold, which may have caused the problem, since boiling usually kills the bacteria and destroys the poison. The soup killed one man and caused grave illness in two others. As a result, all Bon Vivant soups were taken off the shelves by order of the Food and Drug Administration (FDA).

Even though the problem was traced to just one batch of soup, people were reluctant to buy the Bon Vivant brand. Because of what had happened, Bon Vivant had to destroy one million cans of perfectly safe soup. Recognizing that the damage to its brand name was beyond repair, Bon Vivant Soups changed its name to Moore & Co.

Trini & Carmen's Hot Sauce

In 1974, nacho sauce produced by a Pontiac, Michigan, restaurant called Trini & Carmen's was the cause of a well-known botulism incident in the United States. Trini and Carmen Martinez, the owners of the Mexican restaurant, used home-canning methods to preserve their nacho hot sauce. No one died in this incident, but fifty-nine people became very ill. Unlike Bon Vivant, though, the Trini & Carmen name survived the bad publicity. A chain of Trini & Carmen's restaurants is still in business in the Midwest.

4

TYPES OF BOTULISM

Scientists now classify botulism into seven types: A, B, C, D, E, F, and G. Types A, B, E, and F mainly affect human beings. These are all forms of the same bacteria, *C. botulinum*. Types C and D affect wild birds and poultry, cattle, horses, turtles, sheep, and some species of fish. Types A and B are the types commonly found in most botulism outbreaks, while type A is the deadliest form of them all.

There are four kinds of human botulism known today. The first discovered form, which is also the best known, is foodborne botulism, or botulism caused by eating contaminated food. Doctors and public health officials have been on the alert for this type of botulism ever since the outbreaks of the early twentieth century. There

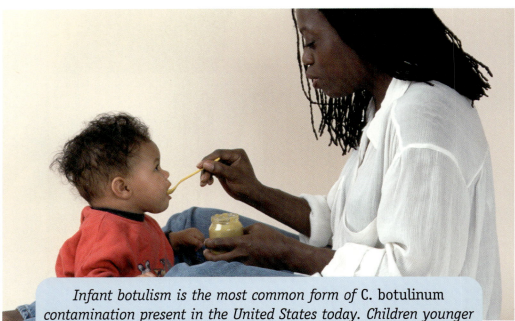

Infant botulism is the most common form of C. botulinum *contamination present in the United States today. Children younger than one year old are particularly susceptible to the bacteria.*

have been around a thousand outbreaks of foodborne botulism in the last hundred years.

Infant Botulism

The most common kind of botulism reported in the United States today affects only babies. Called infant botulism, the disease occurs when a baby under one year of age swallows food that contains *C. botulinum* spores. Once inside the baby's intestinal tract, the bacteria grow and produce the deadly botulinum toxin.

C. botulinum spores are very widespread in nature. In fact, older children and adults swallow them all the time without experiencing any ill effects, since the spores are destroyed by the body's chemicals. Infants, however, have not yet developed these chemicals, which is why they are so vulnerable to infection.

Surprisingly, about 20 percent of the cases of infant botulism are caused by spores that have been found in honey. As a result, public health officials now warn parents against feeding honey to children who are under twelve months old.

Although infant botulism has always been around, doctors did not become aware of the problem until 1976. Some believe that many of the unexplained deaths that are attributed to sudden infant death syndrome (SIDS), or crib death, which is a mysterious cause of death among infants, were in fact misdiagnosed cases of infant botulism.

Wound Botulism

Wounds are vulnerable to getting infected with *C. botulinum*. But wounds are usually protected from infection because they are usually bathed in blood, which is rich in the oxygen that kills *C. botulinum*. For this reason, wound botulism is a rare form of the

Though wound botulism was reported much earlier, cases were scarce until the early 1990s, when doctors in California began noticing a sharp rise in this rare form of the disease. All of these cases occurred in California among drug addicts using a dark and gummy substance known as black tar heroin.

Black tar heroin is made secretly in Mexico near the places where opium poppies are grown. Like other illegal drugs, black tar heroin is mixed in with other substances to give the appearance of there being more of the drug than there actually is. That way there's more of it to sell, and the sellers can make more money. But in addition to diluting

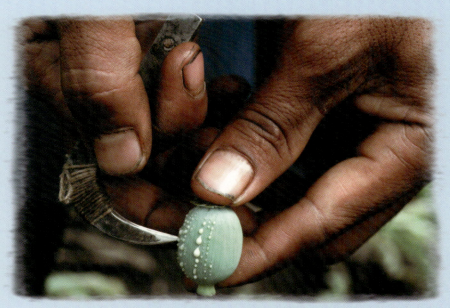

An opium harvester cuts open an opium poppy, which black tar heroin is made from. Using illegal drugs intravenously can lead to cases of wound botulism.

the product, mixing other substances into it increases the chance that it will be contaminated with impurities such as *C. botulinum* spores.

Physicians cannot be sure as to the exact cause of this kind of botulism. When *C. botulinum* is found in a can of olives or a tub of chili, public health authorities can easily check every stage of manufacture to find out what caused the problem. But when a drug that is being illegally manufactured and secretly sold causes botulism, the mystery is a lot harder to solve.

In the meantime, public health authorities have spread the word to doctors to be on the lookout for cases of wound botulism. Just as botulism should be suspected when someone shows symptoms of the disease after eating a home-canned food, it should be suspected when someone with the symptoms of botulism is a drug addict of some kind.

Doctors are trying to get the word out to the addicts. A Web page sponsored by the San Francisco Department of Health warns illegal drug users of the risk of contracting botulism if they take their drugs intravenously.

disease. In severe injuries, however, some tissues can die, therefore becoming free of oxygen. Once free of oxygen, the tissues give the *C. botulinum* spores the opportunity to become active bacteria. Once active, the bacteria will multiply and produce the botulinum toxin. The victims of this form of botulism usually suffer from symptoms such as muscle weakness and paralysis without the vomiting and nausea that often go with foodborne botulism.

Since doctors first reported a case of wound botulism in 1951, it has been considered a very rare illness. Most of the cases have involved people who had suffered extremely severe injuries. In the 1980s, however, physicians began to notice cases of wound botulism among users of illegal drugs. Some were cocaine users who had developed sores in their nostrils or sinuses from snorting the drug. But the majority of the drug users who were coming down with wound botulism were taking their drugs intravenously, using needles. It turned out that it was the needle use that caused them to contract the disease. By continuously puncturing their skin with needles, the heroin addicts were giving themselves a number of small wounds. After puncturing the same wound over and over again, the wound would turn into dead tissue, which provided the kind of oxygen-free environment that *C. botulinum* needs to thrive.

Avian Botulism

Botulism doesn't just kill human beings. In fact, human beings are far less likely to fall victim to botulism than are some animals. For birds in particular, botulism can be a terrible scourge, at times striking millions at once. It is one of the three most serious

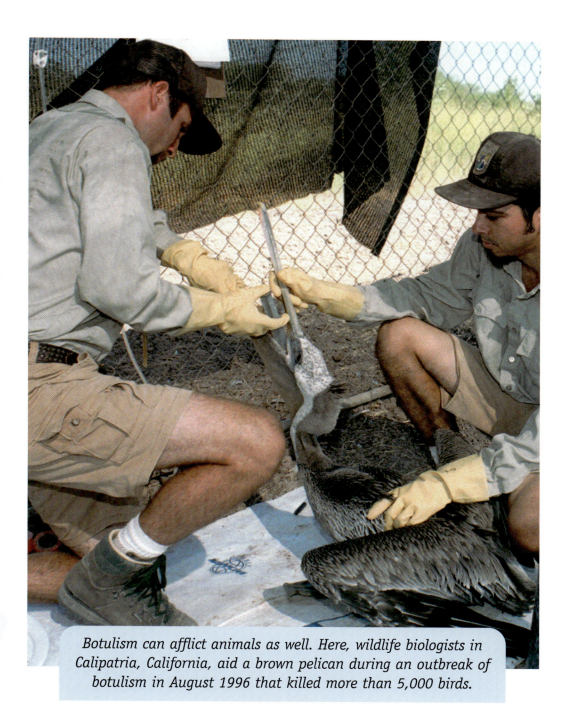

Botulism can afflict animals as well. Here, wildlife biologists in Calipatria, California, aid a brown pelican during an outbreak of botulism in August 1996 that killed more than 5,000 birds.

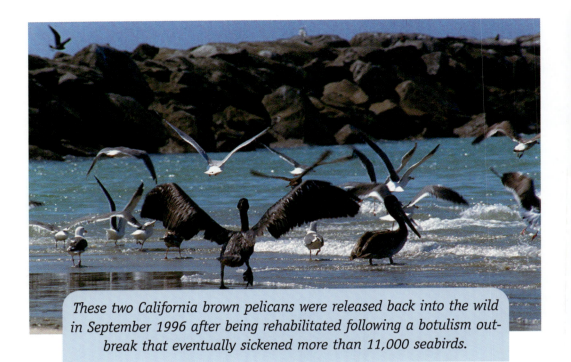

These two California brown pelicans were released back into the wild in September 1996 after being rehabilitated following a botulism outbreak that eventually sickened more than 11,000 seabirds.

disease problems of wild migratory birds, mainly affecting ducks, geese, swans, and shore birds. Due to its prevalence among birds, observers called the disease western duck sickness before it came to be known as avian botulism.

Although the strain of *C. botulinum* that causes avian botulism is different from the strains that harm human beings, the disease is essentially the same. Avian botulism affects the nervous system, causing muscle paralysis. An early sign in birds is the inability to fly. Next, the leg muscles become paralyzed. Ducks suffering from botulism often move across the water with their wings. Then the neck muscles become paralyzed. In fact, the disease is sometimes referred to as "limberneck" because of the infected birds' inability to hold their heads erect. Birds with severe cases of botulism either drown or, like human beings with botulism, die when their muscles become so paralyzed that they are no longer able to breathe.

5

BATTLING BOTULISM

Even with today's medical advances, botulism is still a dangerous and often deadly disease. Fortunately, though, doctors have gotten better at treating its victims. People who contract botulism are much less likely to die than they were only a few decades ago. Between 1910 and 1919, the death rate from botulism was 70 percent. By the 1980s, it had dropped to 9 percent, and by the 1990s, it was only 6 percent. These statistics do not apply to infant botulism, however. Since this form of botulism has only been discovered recently, statistics about it have not yet been compiled.

Since most deaths due to botulism occur when the muscles that control breathing are paralyzed, putting the afflicted person on a breathing machine is an important treatment for the disease. Breathing machines allow people in the later stages of the illness to survive. With good medical care, even victims who have reached this stage of the disease eventually recover fully.

Diagnosis and Treatment

The earlier botulism is caught, the easier it is to treat, so it is important for doctors to recognize it immediately. As with any illness, the patient's symptoms are the first clues. In the case of botulism, the next most important clue is the patient's history, which usually means what foods the person has eaten recently. Doctors can then conduct laboratory tests to look for the toxin in the patient's bloodstream. If the food that is suspected of having caused the botulism is not yet digested, it can be tested as well.

As soon as botulism is suspected, doctors order an antitoxin, which is available in the United States from the CDC. State and local health departments maintain supplies of a "trivalent" botulinum antitoxin. It is called "trivalent" ("tri" means "three") because it contains antibodies for the toxins produced by three different types of *C. botulinum* bacteria— types A, B, and E, the three most common types of the botulism toxin in humans.

The antitoxin stops the action of the poison, preventing further damage from occurring. Since the antitoxin works best when given early, public health officials tell doctors to give it immediately to people who show even the slightest symptoms of botulism.

At the same time, doctors may try to remove whatever contaminated food might still be in the body by inducing vomiting. In the case of wound botulism, physicians use surgery to clean out the wound and kill the bacteria.

Some of the treatments that are given to adults with botulism, however, could actually end up doing more harm than good to babies who have botulism. For example, doctors have found out by experience that the use of antibiotics in cases of infant botulism can backfire, making the babies sicker. Why this happens is not completely known. Scientists suspect it is because for some reason antibiotics activate the *C. botulinum* bacteria that are present in babies' bodies, which results in the bacteria releasing extra toxins when they are killed by the antibiotics.

Doctors have also found that the botulinum antitoxin that helps adults with botulism can make babies who are infected with the disease sicker. A new botulinum antitoxin has been developed to treat babies with botulism. In the late 1990s, it was tested on sick babies, and the results showed that it is safer and more effective.

Preventing Botulism

The most preventable form of botulism is the food-borne kind, and government and industry have been quite successful in preventing outbreaks that are caused by food. Incidents that are the result of commercial canning have dropped dramatically because today canneries are well informed about proper canning methods. Inspections are performed at every stage of the process. This is the result of the hard lessons that the canning industry learned early in the twentieth century.

However, since the government can't send health inspectors into the kitchens of the homes of people who do their own canning, foodborne botulism from home canning is still a problem. Government agencies such as the CDC, the FDA, and the U.S. Department of Agriculture (USDA) provide free information to home canners. To avoid botulism, people canning low-acid foods are advised to use a pressure canner, which allows cans to reach 248°F (120°C), the temperature needed to kill *C. botulinum* spores, without exploding.

Even pressure canners can be dangerous, however, when the gauge of the pressure canner gives a false reading. So home canners should have their gauges checked periodically to make sure that they're working properly. Pressure cookers designed to cook food

Despite the devastation that botulism is known to unleash, botulism can actually be a healer. The key to this dual nature of botulism—as killer and healer—lies in the way that the botulinum toxin acts on muscle nerves. Many serious disorders that human beings are prey to are the result of muscles that contract when they shouldn't. A paralyzing chemical can help people who suffer from these disorders, since it can reduce, or eliminate, these unwanted contractions.

In December 1989, the FDA approved a new form of botulinum toxin for commercial use. The new form of the toxin, which is made from type A botulinum, the strongest and deadliest type, was marketed under the trade name

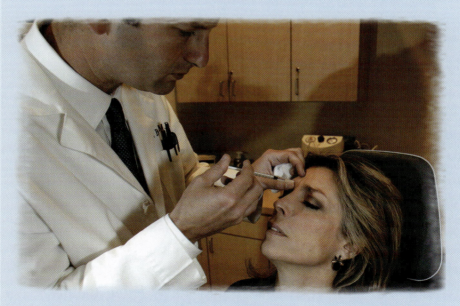

A Philadelphia doctor injects Botox into a patient's face in April 2002 during a cosmetic procedure.

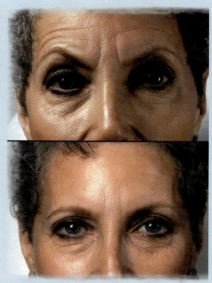

Botox eliminates wrinkles by paralyzing facial muscles.

Botox. Botox works by preventing the muscle from having extra contractions while also leaving it enough strength for normal use.

After its initial approval, the drug began to be used by doctors to treat disorders that involve the cramping of muscles. Botox has eased the muscle contractions of patients with cerebral palsy and has reduced involuntary facial tics. It has helped people who are unable to swallow their food or use their bladders. It has given stroke victims back the use of their clenched and rigid hands. It has even helped people suffering from writer's cramp.

Botulinum toxin has "an amazing safety record," says Bill Habig, Ph.D., former deputy director of the FDA's division of bacterial products in the Center for Biologics Evaluation and Research. Habig says that at first there was a lot of concern about its use, considering the fact that it is one of the most toxic materials around. But after repeated use with no ill effects, that concern has eased.

Even so, officials at the FDA were shocked when they noticed, early in the 1990s, that some doctors were giving Botox injections as a form of beauty treatment. These doctors were using the substance to smooth out wrinkles by

(Continued on page 54)

weakening facial muscles. In 1994, the FDA called this "an egregious example of promoting a potentially toxic biologic for cosmetic purposes." Still, despite its objections to Botox being used for this purpose, the government was not legally able to prevent physicians from giving it to their patients to help them look younger. Botox injections soon became the hottest thing in cosmetic treatments. As it turns out, the treatments, which cost approximately $600 each and last for four to six months, have proven to be safe. In April 2002, the FDA reluctantly gave its approval to the cosmetic use of Botox.

quickly can also be used in home canning. In this case also, it's important to get the gauges checked.

When canning food that is low in acid, it is wise to boil the food for ten minutes before it's eaten. Even when botulinum toxin is present in the food, ten minutes of boiling will neutralize the toxin.

Finding Botulism

When a patient comes into a doctor's office suffering from foodborne botulism, it becomes a public health emergency since the source of the illness could still be lurking somewhere outside the doctor's office. Each case of botulism presents a mystery that calls for a quick solution. Was the cause a food? If so, where is it and where are the people who ate it?

Each state in the United States has a list of notifiable conditions, illnesses that must be reported to the health department. Diagnosed cases of serious infections are routinely reported to the CDC. Tens of thousands of cases of these notifiable conditions are reported every year.

The immediate task of finding the culprit is the job of local health departments. In most cases, the outbreaks are small. The causes of the contamination are usually foods prepared in a home or at a restaurant. The local health department can search for the toxic food and round up potential victims who might be in need of medical treatment. In the case of a very large or unusual outbreak, the CDC may send a team into the field to help state public health officials conduct emergency investigations.

The CDC usually helps local health departments in a more general way, acting as a clearinghouse for information about botulism outbreaks, conducting research, and providing expert advice as needed. CDC researchers develop new methods for identifying the microbes that cause disease.

C. botulinum bacteria and spores are so widespread in nature that we'll probably never be able to completely eradicate them. One advantage we have, though, is that we've learned an amazing amount about botulism. By applying what we've come to know, human beings can retain the upper hand in our battle against this deadly enemy.

GLOSSARY

anaerobic   Living, acting, or occurring in the absence of free oxygen.

bacteria   Extremely small one-celled organisms that usually have a cell wall and multiply by cell division.

Clostridium botulinum (C. botulinum)   A spore-forming bacterium that produces a powerful nerve poison.

egregious   Conspicuous or flagrant.

foodborne   Spread by means of food.

outbreak   A sudden rise in the incidence of a disease.

scavenger   An organism that feeds habitually on refuse or dead meat.

scourge   A cause of widespread or great affliction.

spore An inactive form taken by a bacterium when it dries out and forms a tough husk.

sterilize To deprive of the power of reproducing or to free from living organisms.

strain A group of organisms of the same species possessing distinctive hereditary characters that distinguish them from other such groups.

toxin Poison.

FOR MORE INFORMATION

In the United States

Centers for Disease Control and Prevention (CDC)
1600 Clifton Road
Atlanta, GA 30333
(404) 639-3311
(800) 311-3435
Web site: http://www.cdc.gov

National Institutes of Health (NIH)
9000 Rockville Pike
Bethesda, MD 20892
(301) 496-4000
Web site: http://www.nih.gov/health/infoline.htm

In Canada

Health Canada
Suite 1802, 18th Floor, Maritime Centre
1505 Barrington Street
Halifax, NS B3J 3Y6
(902) 426-2700
Web site: http://www.hc-sc.gc.ca

Web Sites

Due to the changing nature of Internet links, the Rosen Publishing Group, Inc., has developed an online list of Web sites related to the subject of this book. This site is updated regularly. Please use this link to access the list:

http://www.rosenlinks.com/epid/botu

FOR FURTHER READING

Altman, Linda Jacobs. *Plague and Pestilence: A History of Infectious Disease*. New York: Enslow Publishers, Inc., 1998.

Desalle, Rob. *Epidemic! The World of Infectious Disease*. New York: The New Press, 1999.

Farrell, Jeannette. *Invisible Enemies: Stories of Infectious Disease*. New York: Farrar Straus & Giroux, 1998.

Friedlander, Mark P., and Leonard T. Kurland. *Outbreak: Disease Detectives at Work*. New York: Lerner Publications Company, 2000.

Lemaster, Leslie Jean. *Bacteria and Viruses*. New York: Children's Press, 1999.

Marsh, Carole. *Hot Zones: Disease, Epidemics, Viruses & Bacteria*. Peachtree City, GA: Gallopade Publishing Group, 1997.

Young, Lisa. *Disease Detectives*. New York: Lucent Books, 2000.

INDEX

CREDITS

About the Author

Maxine Rosaler is a freelance writer who lives in New York City.

Photo Credits

Cover and chapter title interior photos, p. 15 © A. B. Dowsett/SPL/Custom Medical Stock Photo; p. 4 © SuperStock; p. 9 © Ludovic Maisant/Corbis; p. 13 © Bettmann/Corbis; p. 17 © U.S. Fish and Wildlife Service/Image Collection; p. 27 © National Archives/Timepix; p. 29 © Chikumo Chiaki/AP/Wide World Photos; p. 31 © William Gottlieb/Corbis; p. 34 © Hulton-Deutsch Collection/Corbis; p. 40 © Jennie Woodcock/Reflections Photolibrary/Corbis; p. 42 © Michael Freeman/Corbis; p. 45 © Michael Poche/Corbis; p. 46 © Reed Saxon/Corbis; p. 52 © Getty Images; p. 53 © Tannen Maury/The Image Works.

Designer: Evelyn Horovicz; Editor: Nicholas Croce